PRAISE FOR Q's ENCORE METHOD FROM FORMER CLIENTS:

"QUINCY'S CORE EXERCISES are unique and translate all over my body and within my athletic play."- **Emily R.**

"I HAVE BEEN TRAINING with Quincy since high school, and his core methods have prepared me for success as a Division I lacrosse player. The change in my inner core strength has taken my abilities to the next level as a competitive athlete. This strength gives me a powerful shot and a strong defensive stance. By following his routines, I have seen dramatic change in my power and ability in all of my physical activities. I feel great and look great! I will always recommend Quincy's core routines to any person that wants to improve their core strength. If you are seeking real and lasting results that surpass typical core exercises, this is your book!" - **Chloe P.**

"AS PARENTS OF THREE highly competitive student-athletes, we are confident their strength and development will benefit from Quincy's workout routines. From sport-specific and very focused training to prepare them for time on the basketball courts, football fields, and in the swimming pools, to encouraging a love of competition and creating mental toughness, Quincy is a significant role model and leader as they continue to develop and grow. **Q's ENCORE** workout is challenging them to push limits and break boundaries in a healthy, active way, led by the best!" - Parents of Columbus Academy Vikings (Class of '25,'27,'29) **M. Chance Spalding**, DO, PhD, FACS and **E. Spalding**

"AS A HIGH SCHOOL ATHLETE transitioning to a highly competitive Division I swim program, I wanted to prepare myself physically and mentally for the aggressive training regimen required of a collegiate student athlete. I added an enhanced strength and conditioning program working with Quincy 2-3 times per week in order to take my athletic performance to the next level. Quincy's targeted **Q's ENCORE METHOD** workouts completely changed my body in just six months' time. My before- and after-body scan statistics say it all - I decreased my body fat by 3% in my arms, 5% in my legs and 12% in my torso, all while increasing my body's overall lean muscle by 5%! Quincy's emphasis on core and targeted muscle groups immediately impacted my endurance and strength in the water, which was reflected in my improved times. My confidence increased significantly, as did my capacity to push myself harder… Quincy's workouts made an immediate impact on my mindset, drive, and commitment to being the best collegiate athlete that I can be." - **Sydney B.**

"LET ME TELL YOU MY STORY about how this core strength book completely transformed my fitness journey. Whether I was at the gym, participating in sports, or simply working out at home, this book was the ultimate game-changer. The 7 Levels of the **Q's ENCORE METHOD** provided me with a clear path to success, emphasizing body positioning, stability, control, and proper breathing techniques. As an athlete, I found that my performance improved drastically as I strengthened my core. It wasn't just about having a strong physique; it was about unlocking my body's true potential to move efficiently and powerfully. This book became my constant companion, guiding me toward my goals and pushing me to new heights. Whether you're an athlete, a gym enthusiast, or someone who loves to exercise at home, trust me, this book will greatly benefit you. It's time to rewrite your fitness story and unleash the incredible power of your core muscles." - **C. Baron**

LINK CORE MUSCLES:
Q's ENCORE METHOD

BY ODIS QUINCY KIDD III

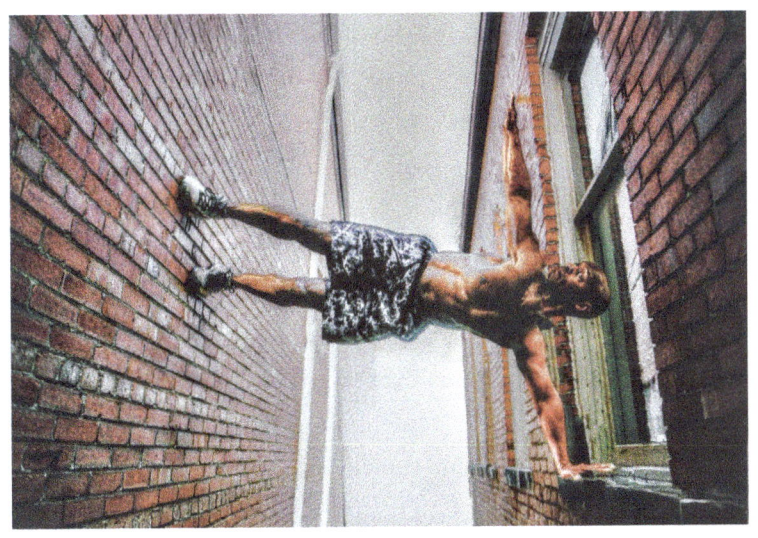

QUINCY, BRIDGING THE GAP TO SUCCESS

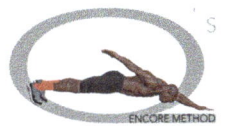

Copyright © 2025 by Odis Quincy Kidd III

All rights reserved. No part of this publication, *Link Core Muscles: Q's ENCORE METHOD*, may be reproduced, distributed, or transmitted in any form or by any means, including photocopying, recording, or other electronic or mechanical methods, without the prior written permission of the author, except in the case of brief quotations embodied in critical reviews and certain other noncommercial uses permitted by copyright law.

Paperback ISBN: 978-1-63337-926-8
eBook ISBN: 978-1-63337-927-5

Disclaimer: The information provided in this book is for educational and informational purposes only. The author and publisher are not responsible for any actions taken based on the information contained in this book.

I DEDICATE THIS BOOK TO
THE CITY OF NEW ALBANY, OHIO AND ITS
PASSIONATE FITNESS COMMUNITY.

Q's ENCORE METHOD (Q's EM)
10 MOTIVATING MESSAGES

1. Calling all parents! If your child needs to improve athleticism in their chosen sport, **Q's ENCORE METHOD** is the ultimate game-changer to give them the winning edge.

2. For middle school, high school, college, or aspiring pro-level athletes, **Q's ENCORE METHOD** is a must-have book consisting of highly accessible, robust guidance that will revolutionize your athleticism and enhance body control like never before.

3. Gain that competitive advantage you've been seeking **with Q's ENCORE METHOD** book, which provides essential techniques for improving body control and optimizing movement at every level of play.

4. Unlock the secrets of athleticism with **Q's ENCORE METHOD** book, which can be specifically helpful to parents who want to see their child's performance soar in their sport of play.

5. Elevate your game to new heights! **Q's ENCORE METHOD** guarantees giving you the edge you need in boosting body control and enhancing movement, regardless of your skill level.

6. Whether your child is playing recreational sports or aiming for the professional level, **Q's ENCORE METHOD** book is the ultimate resource for parents who want to help their young athletes develop superior body control and movement skills.

7. Stand out above your competitors! The **ENCORE METHOD** book, developed by '**Q**', provides in-depth mind-focus guidance and practical techniques to improve your body control and movement. This resource enables you to excel in any sport or physical activity, promoting explosive body reaction time and increasing endurance.

8. Ranging from foundational exercises to advanced training strategies, **Q's ENCORE METHOD** book covers the entire spectrum of athleticism, including individuals of all levels, from middle school up to pro-level athletes. Even if you are already a physically active person we have you covered.

9. Give your child or yourself the gift of improved athleticism with **Q's ENCORE METHOD** book. These essential resources are designed to provide a comprehensive blueprint for boosting body control and refining movement patterns.

10. Embrace the game-changing power of **Q's ENCORE METHOD** book and witness the incredible progress your body will make from these 7 Levels. These motivating messages offer invaluable insights and techniques to master body control and unlock the true potential of movement.

UNDERSTANDING AND FOLLOWING THE 7 LEVELS EXPLAINED IN THIS BOOK ARE THE KEYS TO HOW YOUR BODY ADAPTS TO EVERYDAY AND ATHLETIC DEMANDS.

MY MISSION

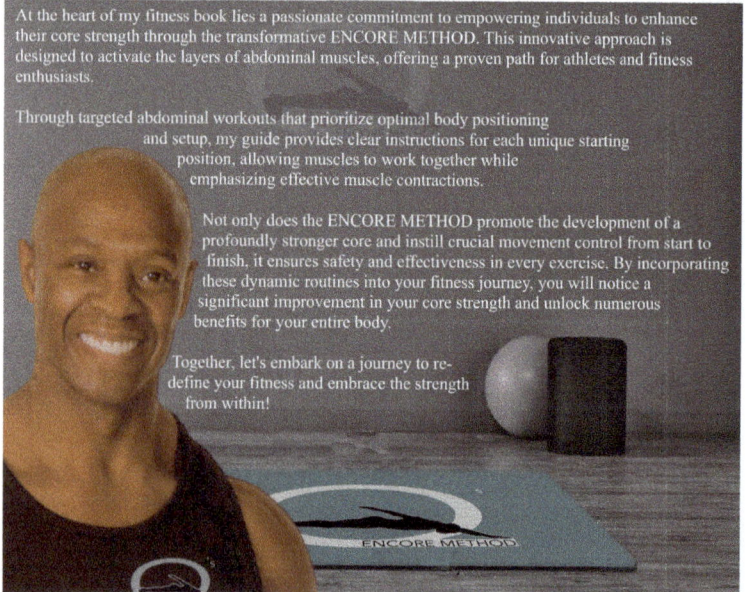

At the heart of my fitness book lies a passionate commitment to empowering individuals to enhance their core strength through the transformative ENCORE METHOD. This innovative approach is designed to activate the layers of abdominal muscles, offering a proven path for athletes and fitness enthusiasts.

Through targeted abdominal workouts that prioritize optimal body positioning and setup, my guide provides clear instructions for each unique starting position, allowing muscles to work together while emphasizing effective muscle contractions.

Not only does the ENCORE METHOD promote the development of a profoundly stronger core and instill crucial movement control from start to finish, it ensures safety and effectiveness in every exercise. By incorporating these dynamic routines into your fitness journey, you will notice a significant improvement in your core strength and unlock numerous benefits for your entire body.

Together, let's embark on a journey to redefine your fitness and embrace the strength from within!

DISCLAIMER: Before starting this exercise program, please consult with your doctor and seek medical advice regarding any injuries, especially if you are experiencing back-related injuries or pain.

TABLE OF CONTENTS

About the Author i

Introduction iii

Chapter 1: Learning About the Core Muscles 1

Chapter 2: Q's ENCORE METHOD and
Progress Chart 11

Chapter 3: Q's ENCORE METHOD 21

Chapter 4: Putting Q's ENCORE METHOD
into Action 45

Bonus Section: Q Recommends Three
Essential Core Stretches 47

Conclusion 53

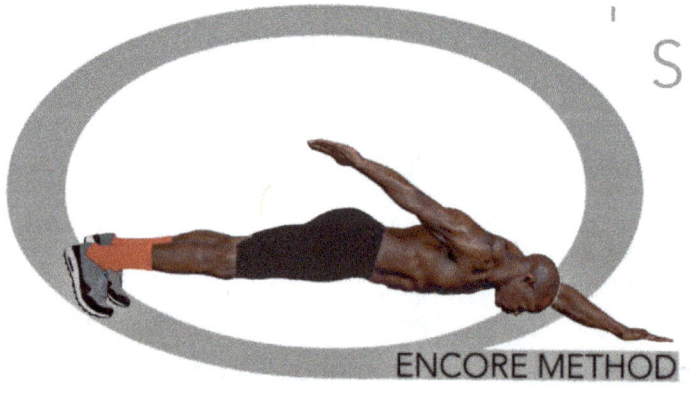

ABOUT THE AUTHOR

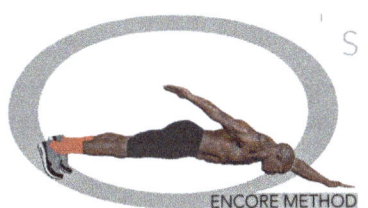

ODIS QUINCY KIDD III, who goes by Quincy or 'Q', is an expert in his field of Personal Training. He understands on a deep level how important it is to be healthy and fit and brings his enthusiasm and confidence to his clients. He has trained athletes of all levels, from young and inexperienced to elite professionals. Quincy understands the obstacles people face in reaching their goals and makes it his priority to find the best workout program to lead his clients to success.

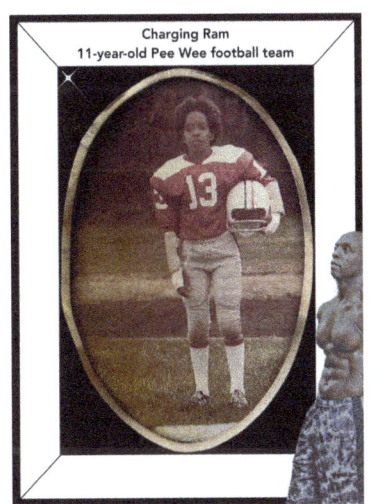

Charging Ram
11-year-old Pee Wee football team

MY YOUTH STORY

I had a number of friends in middle school, several of whom played summer league Pee Wee football. A few of them on the Charging Rams team encouraged me to join because they knew I was competitive and quick on my feet. After rejecting the idea the previous year, my mom finally agreed to let me play. Both my friends and I were thrilled! At age 11, I stepped into the world of sports, a journey that would shape my understanding of competition. Upon meeting my teammates, I quickly noticed that I was the only African American on the team, but it didn't bother me much. As the coaches assessed our skills and assigned positions, I was given the roles of halfback and wide receiver. Happy as I was, I soon realized I was facing an uphill battle.

As I donned my jersey for the first time, a mixture of excitement and anxiety filled me. I loved the idea of playing football, but I couldn't shake the feeling that I was at a disadvantage. Most of my teammates had been playing together for years, and they seemed to possess an innate understanding of the game. I often found myself watching from the sidelines, feeling the sting of disappointment and inadequacy, as I struggled to keep pace with their skills.

Despite my competitive spirit and determination, my lack of experience became glaringly evident. On the field, I felt like I was in a constant race against time, frantically trying to learn plays and techniques while my teammates executed them with confidence. I could mentally visualize the moves I needed to make and understood the strategies, but translating that knowledge into action proved to be more challenging than I had anticipated.

As practices progressed, I realized that my physical readiness wasn't where it needed to be. There were moments when I felt capable and quick in my mind, but physically, I was often left behind. I knew I needed to change that. Sitting on the sidelines, watching my friends play, fueled my desire to improve. I wanted

ABOUT THE AUTHOR | III

to prove to myself, and to my teammates, that I could contribute to the team.

The journey wasn't easy. In Possum Elementary school in Ohio, when I was 11, all I could do were standard at-home physical exercises, like push-ups, jumping jacks, jump rope, and full sit-ups. I even wore ankle weights because I felt I had tried just about everything. I realized that despite all I was doing to get stronger and faster, my teammates had the advantage of years of playing and training that I was lacking. Back then, coaches never had us doing any kind of planks or leg lifts. Pretty much all we ever did were high knee tire foot agility drills, push-ups, and just running up and down the field. Even though in my years at Shawnee High School, I had always maintained my competitiveness and made significant progress, there were still some setbacks along the way. I couldn't figure out how to elevate my game.

After years of weight training, powerlifting, and bodybuilding, I sought out what would take me to a higher level of performance and began to research anatomy and core exercises on my own.

QUINCY IS A Certified Personal Trainer with over 25 years of experience. His additional certifications include **Athletics and Fitness Association of America (AFAA)** and **TRX-Suspension Training**. In the early 1990s Quincy competed in powerlifting. His specialty was the bench press competition and in his 165-pound weight class, he outperformed his competitors and placed first in 11 out of 12 events, the 12th time placing second. His overall max lift was 350lbs. He then got into bodybuilding and competed at an amateur level for three years. After competing in powerlifting and bodybuilding, he was often questioned about his personal routine, his techniques, and his own results. This motivated him to become a Certified Personal Trainer.

He also created a group workout that then turned into a DVD program called **'ROCK-N-ABS' by Q®**, which implemented his unique core moves. Although this DVD is aerobic and core based, it emphasizes overall health and stamina. After teaching **ROCK-N-ABS** classes around Columbus, Ohio, Quincy realized his main goal was to show clients a new, more effective way of positioning the body to enhance core strength. His focus is on core exercises within an aerobic workout to targeted core positioning with an emphasis on whole-body control. He feels these specific core exercises provide a missing key in many people's exercise regimens. After years of researching and crafting his core routine with clients and athletes, Quincy distinguished himself from others in the field with his creation of **Q's ENCORE METHOD**, composed of uniquely positioned and hyper-focused abdominal exercises. And since he can't personally train all who would benefit from these exercises, he wrote this book.

INTRODUCTION

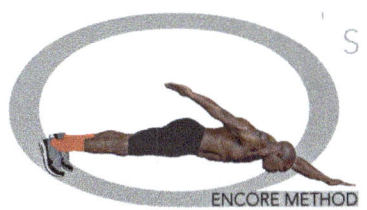

ARE YOU A COLLEGE ATHLETE and want to take your athleticism to a new level? Is your teenager playing at a high intensity and you want to help give them an athletic edge? Or are you someone who wants to improve your own core strength? If so, you have come to the right place. My **Q's ENCORE METHOD** shows you how to tap into your core muscles. My exercises are unique in the way that I isolate and bring attention to the abdominal muscles. Because of the targeted positioning and angles, my **METHOD** leads to a deeper whole-body connection.

This book and my **METHOD** will benefit you whether you are a super-competitive athlete, a long-distance runner, or an avid exerciser looking for something new and different. My **METHOD** has helped many athletes improve their abilities, perform at their best level, and stay ahead of their competitors. I have worked with athletes of all ages for over twenty years, and I can safely say every athlete I have personally trained has noticed a significant change in their athletic careers. **Q's ENCORE METHOD** has given them the tools to achieve success.

Through my observations over the years, I have found many of my clients lack whole-body connection. This disconnect was one of the reasons I was motivated to develop unique core stability exercises. My **METHOD** not only strengthens the core, but it also enables muscle groups to work in unison. By adding my core exercises into your workout routine, you will be able to respond more efficiently during high-intensity movements.

Many things led me to develop this **METHOD,** including my own experience. As a student, I played football, basketball, and ran track & field, which was my favorite sport to play. I had true potential that made recruiters seek me out, but I always felt I was one level below some of my teammates; they received better offers from Division I and II colleges, whereas I had letters from smaller Division II and Division III colleges. *Looking back, I wonder if a strong core was one of the factors that gave them the edge over me.* I had no idea how to engage the right core muscles or how to make them work in unison. My ultimate objective of this book is to help you identify and activate those hidden core muscles. I firmly believe my **METHOD** can unlock that potential hiding within your body and can help you achieve a higher level of performance.

I'd like to present an analogy about the benefit of core strengthening via my **METHOD**. Imagine sitting in your favorite sports car with your helmet on at the Indianapolis Speedway for a four-lap test drive. You slowly drive up to the starting line and the official raises one arm with his palm facing you, telling you to wait - surprisingly, another driver is pulling up next to you in the same exact car. And, as you glance over at the other driver, the official gives both of you the thumbs up to be ready for the green light. Once the light turns green, you both accelerate, and you pull ahead and lead for the first lap.

INTRODUCTION | VII

On the second lap, you stay close to the inside lane, but she passes you on the right side of your car, and while you are on the curve you think, "Wow. That was a very bold move to make. If she can pull that off, I'm going to do the same thing to her on the next lap, on the very same curve." Fast forward, you are now within feet of her bumper, and you decide to duplicate the same bold move on the curve. You end up losing control and your vehicle slides off the track into the grass. You sit there pondering, "Why did I spin out and she didn't?"

Here's the difference: what you didn't realize was that her car was equipped on the inside with a customized high-performance suspension system. From the outside, it looked exactly the same as yours. I would say her "car" went through my **METHOD** and yours did not. You can't always tell from the outside how strong or responsive a person's body is, so my **METHOD** is about unseen strength and connection, not necessarily a change in physique. Let us begin our time together by learning about our core muscle structure and then dig into the specific exercises.

```
LACROSSE   TRACK AND FIELD   FIELD HOCKEY   WEIGHTLIFTING
FOOTBALL   TENNIS   BASKETBALL   CYCLING   SPEED SKATING
BASEBALL   SURFING   GYMNASTICS   SOFTBALL   CHORES AT HOME
SOCCER   FIGURE SKATING   WRESTLING   HIKING   PHYSICAL JOBS
SKIING   SNOWBOARDING   ICE HOCKEY   SWIMMING   FENCING
CHEERLEADING   MOTOCROSS   SKY DIVING   VOLLEYBALL
PICKLEBALL   RUGBY   WALKING   POSTURE   ARCHERY
ROCK CLIMBING   RUNNING   ROWING   COMBAT SPORTS
```

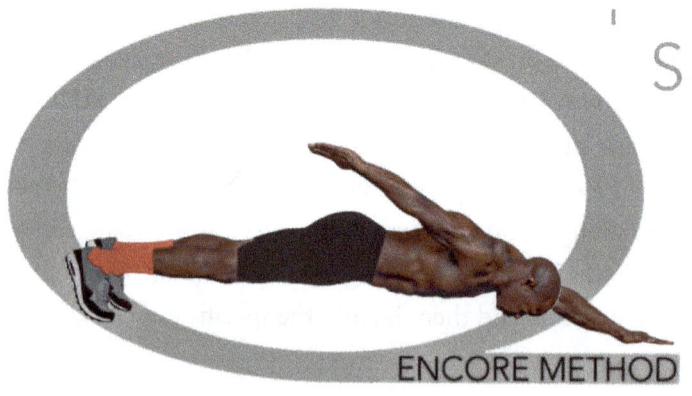

1.
LEARNING ABOUT THE CORE MUSCLES

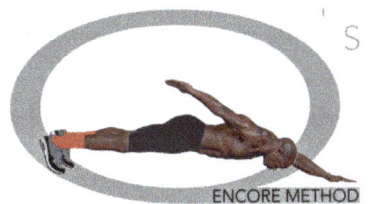

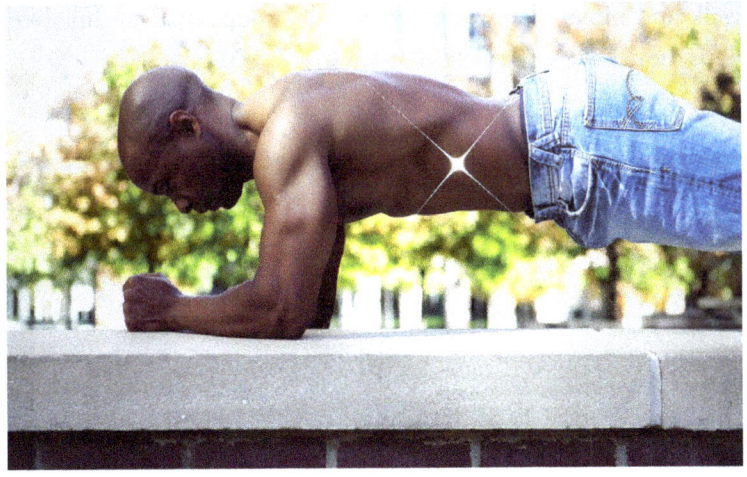

AS I STUDIED AND DUG deeper into my field, I was fascinated to learn more about muscle structure. For the purpose of this book, I'm going to focus on the specific muscle groups that will enhance the body and its ability to adapt to functional movement and athletic challenges. With this information, I thought about how to maximize the working muscles. This thought led me to create the unique positions and angles of my **ENCORE METHOD** exercises. After helping numerous clients through my **METHOD**, I kept getting feedback about an additional benefit. Clients would tell me, "Quincy, when I'm in the game, I just feel better and it's like I can stay longer in the zone." Others reported, "My body just responds more naturally without me having to think about how I'm going to react."

After considering these clients' reports and doing some research, I became intent on increasing people's "mind-body connection." That became the foundation of my **METHOD**. The core includes many muscles that function to support the way we walk and move. Below see the muscle groups that are involved with the 7 Levels of **Q's ENCORE METHOD**.

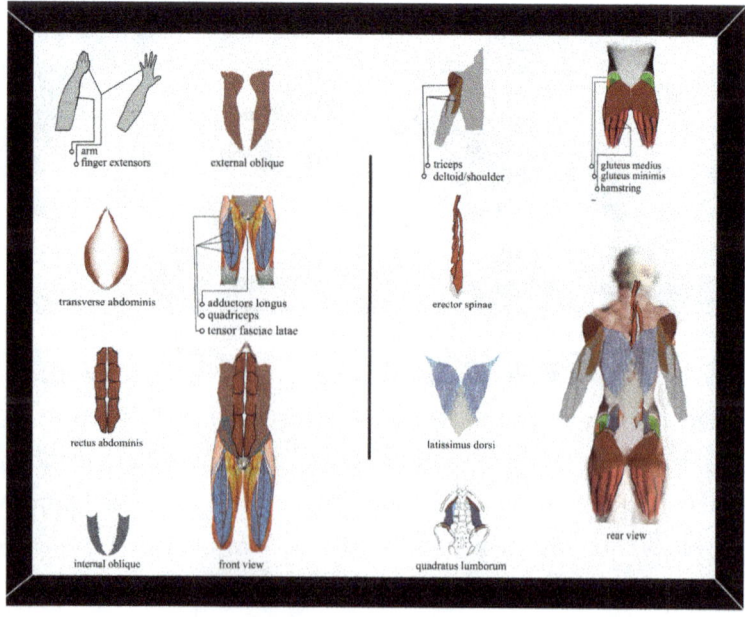

ALL MUSCLE GROUPS INVOLVED IN THE 7 LEVELS

Throughout the book, we are going to primarily focus on the transverse abdominis, external oblique, internal oblique, rectus abdominis, triceps, and deltoid, and to a lesser extent, the latissimus dorsi, quadratus lumborum, hip flexor, and erector spinae group. The core is composed of as many as 35 different muscle groups connecting into the pelvis from the spine and hip area. Additional muscles will provide a supporting role in maintaining the core's movement or static hold, depending on the exercise. But for brevity, it is not necessary to list all muscles involved in each exercise. Instead, we will focus on the primary muscles involved in my **METHOD**.

When I talk about "underlying core muscles" I am referring to muscles that align with the rectus abdominis. These are the most readily recognized of the abdominal muscles. The rectus abdominis runs vertically and along the midline on either side of your belly button. But there is more to our abdominals than just the rectus abdominis. We have muscles that help us twist and turn; those are called the external and internal obliques. The muscle fibers of the external oblique run diagonally, the internal oblique lies underneath, and the fibers run in opposing directions. Beneath the obliques and rectus abdominis lie the transverse abdominis. The fibers run horizontally and are the innermost layer of abdominal muscles. Location and direction of the fibers determine the flexibility of the body's movement.

There is a lot of detail in the setup and instructions for my **METHOD**, but I promise, *with effort and attention to each exercise, the payoff will be HUGE.* You will not only get stronger, but with the extra attention to mirror the exercise you will also see improvement in core strength, body control, and whole-body awareness.

Over the years, gym gurus (in great physical shape) and high-achieving athletes have approached me with questions about my exercises, with them ultimately wanting to give an exercise or two a try. When they tried some of my **Q's ENCORE METHOD** exercises, few were able to complete the moves as instructed despite their physique. Their responses: "I have never felt my core being challenged in such a way - that's amazing!" Initially, these interactions surprised me because these people appeared to be in top physical shape, but the more I observed and taught my **METHOD**, the more I realized how often there can be a disconnect, regardless of appearance. My **METHOD** drew more attention to how core muscles need to work together to hold the unique position of the exercises. It also demonstrated that their muscles were not working in synergy.

Additionally, as I have watched my clients participate in their chosen sports, I noticed that at times their game play falls short of their abilities. They seem to lose body control. Now I'm not talking about complete loss of control, but it seems as if fatigue takes over and they lose the finesse they are known for at their highly competitive level of play. This fatigue is not necessarily indicative of how in shape they are; it could be their core strength is failing them at this point in the game or match. I call it a disconnect. Therefore, one of the main objectives of **Q's ENCORE METHOD** is to teach them to gain body awareness.

Not only will game performance improve as you progress through my book, it will also improve actions you do in everyday life. Having a strong core benefits things we do on a daily basis – walking, reaching for items on a shelf, carrying boxes/kids/pets, gardening, emptying the dishwasher – all things that require our core muscles. But if the core muscles are not working in unison, we are more at risk for an injury. I want to emphasize that my **METHOD** is not only for athletes. I believe a strong core can assist and protect our bodies in everyday life. My exercises target all layers of the core muscles, and in doing so, will help your core and your body function as one.

Studies have also verified additional benefits of core strengthening:

- Strong core muscles help you carry out the toughest physical activities. Weak core muscles often lead to fatigue, less endurance capability, and make you more susceptible to injuries (core muscle disconnect).
- Core muscle training not only strengthens but also improves your mental awareness and balance when engaged in physical activity (link core muscles).
- With repetition and practice you develop muscle memory. This brain-body connection occurs when you repeat the exact exercise routine over and over. This effort and concentration will pay off with correct and efficient muscle firing. Thus, in a game situation, your core will naturally activate effortlessly to give you that competitive edge over your opponents (*turn your muscles on autopilot*).

WARMING UP

Most people try to "rep it out," doing the movement too quickly, thinking that is the best way to get through the routine. But by focusing on form and isolating specific muscle groups through slow, controlled movements, you will see quicker results, improve overall strength, and reduce your risk of injury. Grab a mat, or lie on a padded surface, and let's go!

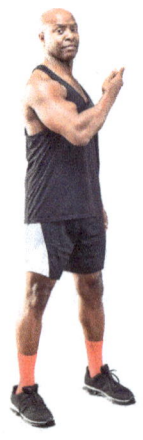

(Please wear comfortable shoes to work out in. Proper foot support is essential to performing my exercises correctly.)

The purpose of a warm-up routine is to loosen your joints, increase blood flow to the muscles, and raise your body temperature. This pre-workout activity helps reduce risk of injury and fatigue later in the workout. The central concept behind my warm-up is to make sure you energize all targeted muscle groups before beginning **Q's ENCORE METHOD**. This warm-up will take approximately five to six minutes. Let's get moving!

> **Discipline forms the foundation upon which success is built**

STANDING CROSSOVER HIGH KNEE

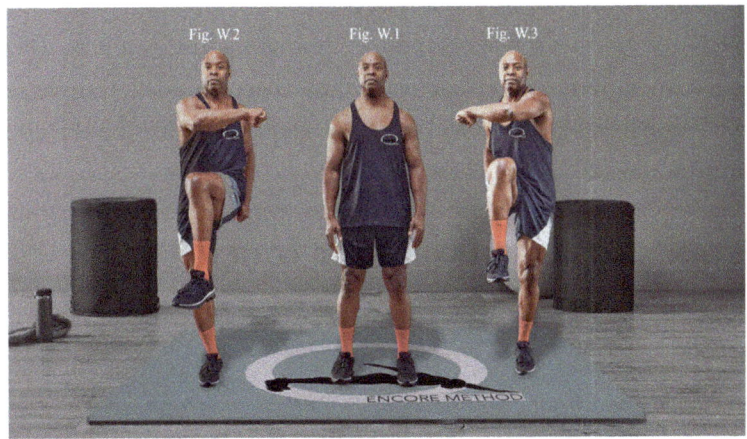

Start with 12 reps of Standing Crossover High Knees. To do this, begin as shown in Fig. W.1. Alternate the left knee to the right elbow, both moving toward the midline of the body for 12 reps (Fig. W.2). As shown in Fig. W.3, you will switch sides, driving the right knee towards the left elbow for another 12 reps. Since this is a warm-up, there is no need to elevate your knee higher than your belly button or to over-rotate. As you elevate your knee and elbow toward your midline, exhale. Inhale as you return to the starting position.

    Next, we are going to replicate the previous movement but this time, alternate right knee raise and then left knee raise to count as one rep. We are going to do 12 reps total. You'll need to modify your breath pattern to shorter inhales and exhales to keep pace with the rotations. Exhale as your elbow and knee move towards your midline. In this warm-up the following muscles are involved: hip flexor, internal, external obliques, deltoid and rectus abdominis muscles.

Now, are you ready to FIRE UP THE CORE? We will complete the warm-up with Standing Alternating Toe Touches. This effective movement will activate those deep, hidden transverse abdominal muscles and will mentally prepare you for the exercise routine ahead … LET'S DO IT!

STANDING ALTERNATING TOE TOUCH

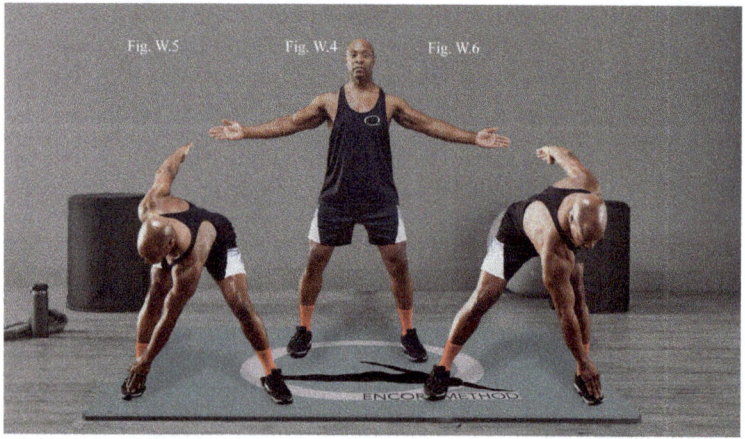

This is one of the most basic, but often overlooked, warm-ups. This stimulates the transverse abdominals, obliques, mid to lower back, glutes, shoulders, latissimus dorsi, hamstrings, and quadriceps muscles.

Do this exercise by standing with your legs apart, greater than shoulder-width, and your arms spread open as shown in Fig. W.4 above. Stand with your legs slightly bent to reduce stress on your lower back to avoid over-stretching your hamstrings. Be sure your knees and toes are pointed slightly away from the midline of the body. Stand all the way up (your full height) before extending your arms down to the opposite side. You should be able to complete all 12 repetitions in 45-60 seconds. As shown in Figs. W.5 and W.6 start with a slow exhale through the rotation of the downward movement. Inhale when returning to the upright position and exhale again as you begin rotating to the opposite side. This completes one rep.

Having completed the warm-up, we are now ready to begin **Q's ENCORE METHOD**, and as I always tell my clients, "Be ready to bring your A-GAME!"

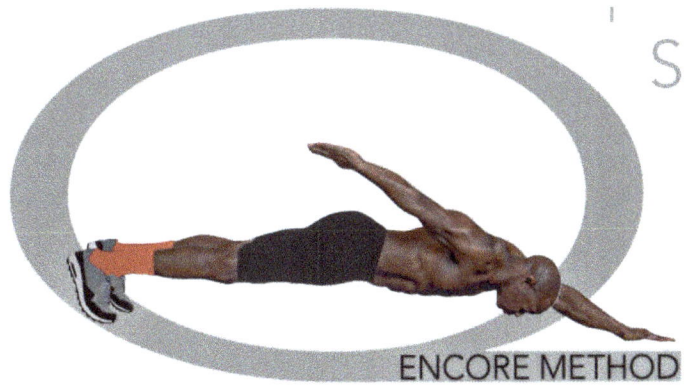

REGARDLESS of whether you're playing offense or defense, you have the opportunity to experience an invigorating feeling as you unlock your body's full potential. The **Q's ENCORE METHOD** is designed to enhance your physical capabilities, allowing you to move with agility, precision, and confidence.

2.
Q's ENCORE METHOD AND PROGRESS CHART

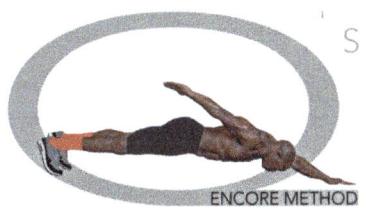

NOW YOU ARE READY to test your focus, body positioning, balance, and control, and put the purpose of this book into action!

Before starting **Q's ENCORE METHOD**, ensure you are hydrated and eat something healthy. I recommend something small and light on the stomach (for example, a serving of yogurt or a small handful of almonds) thirty minutes or more before initiating my routine. Now that it's "go time," keep your water bottle and towel nearby.

These exercises may be difficult when starting, but your core will get stronger, and your body will adapt to the movements with practice. The order of the exercises and the number of repetitions are important. The routine is structured to increase in difficulty and complexity. Doing the levels consecutively will also increase your endurance.

Let's begin here, going through an explanation of the Progress Chart and how to use it. You will familiarize yourself with each Level's positions and begin to practice them.

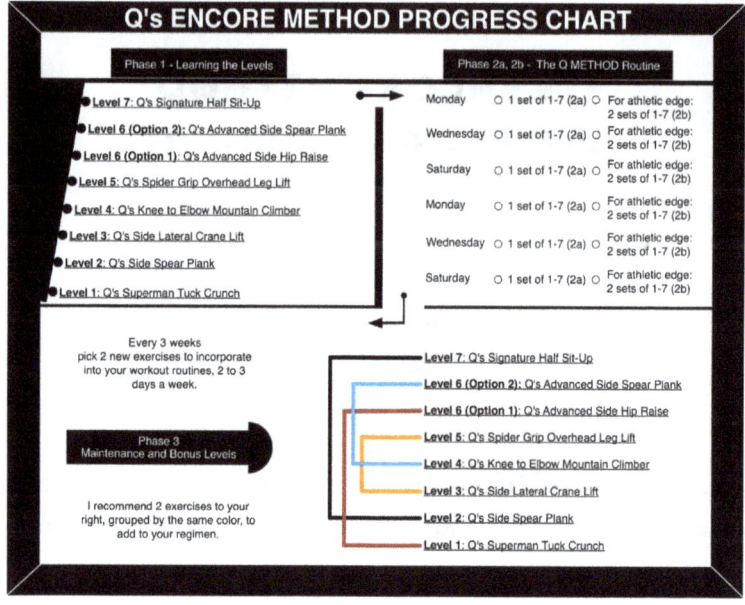

MY METHOD IS BROKEN DOWN INTO THREE PHASES:

- PHASE 1 - LEARNING THE LEVELS—This is where you learn and perfect the movements. It's important not to skip the first phase as jumping straight to the second phase will set you up for failure. Take your time and learn the first phase and you will have a better or higher success rate of finishing the mastery phase.

- PHASE 2A - Q METHOD ROUTINE—Here, you'll do one round of Levels 1-7. This phase is for avid fitness enthusiasts and those working to improve their core strength.

—OR—

- **PHASE 2B - Q METHOD ROUTINE**—This is designed for high-achieving, competitive athletes who want to perform at a higher athletic level. In this phase, you do two rounds of Levels 1-7 in one workout for a total of six sets in two weeks.
- **PHASE 3 - MAINTENANCE AND BONUS**—This is where you incorporate two levels into your current workout routine.

FURTHER EXPLANATION OF PHASES

PHASE 1:

To be successful in this first phase you must always apply these 3 key words:

- Positioning
- Balance
- Control

Keep these at the forefront of your mind when reading my instructions, looking at the images, and noting the angle of my body. Once you're able to focus on each level with those three words in mind, you are well on your way to success.

Another important factor is practicing one level at a time

and in sequence. Go over that specific level until you can maintain control throughout each level. Please make this fun! If you need an extra set of eyes, grab a family member or friend to watch you demonstrate each level. They can give you hands-on assistance to guide you in the movement or help you with balance. Use this assistance until you feel your body is in the right position. You can progress to the next level when you are comfortable with that level and can complete each level without assistance.

My goal for you during the learning phase is to have fun while you practice at each level. Even though you must nail down the specifics of form, angle, balance, and control in addition to coordinating the movement with your breath, I hope you approach my **METHOD** with a positive attitude and determination. This fitness program might be challenging for many, but just like learning your position in your sport of play, repetitions are key. The goal of Phase 1 is to complete all levels as described without losing control or balance and completing all required reps (or static holds). If you cannot complete the level without loss of balance or rest breaks:

1. Stop.
2. Work on that level until you can complete it as described with all the reps, without loss of balance, and with proper form throughout.
3. Regardless of the level that you may find difficult, after completing #2 above, you must begin back at Level 1 and then progress through the levels consecutively.

Once you can complete all seven levels without loss of balance or rest breaks, you are ready for Phase 2a. With that achievement,

Q'S ENCORE METHOD AND PROGRESS CHART | 15

you will have worked to gain confidence and control in each level and be more mentally prepared for Phase 2a. The main differences between Phase 1 and Phase 2a are:

- In Phase 1, you can take your time and test your body's ability while learning these exercises.
- In Phase 2a, you are executing these levels to perfection. Be sure that before moving to Phase 2a, you do not need verbal cues or hands-on assistance. If you want someone to evaluate your movements, however, that is ok.

OKAY (awesome and great job)! Now that you have successfully maintained full body control of all seven levels, IT'S TIME TO TAKE ON Q's NEXT PHASE!

PHASE 2A:

This is the phase where each level needs to be perfected and there are certain criteria for progressing to the next level. This phase is designed to improve what you mastered in Phase 1.

In Phase 2a you must:

1. Replicate the starting point and end point as shown in the images.
2. Control the movement as described.
3. Complete the required number of repetitions.
4. Have no loss of balance (specifics will be listed at each level).
5. Take only a 30-second break between levels in Phase 2a.

Regardless of what group you considered yourself in, you MUST remain focused on the position of your body while bringing your A-GAME!

In addition to perfecting the movement of each level, you must also manage your break time well to succeed in the challenge of Phase 2a. After completing each level there will be a 30-second break. If you need a drink or to wipe off a little sweat, use your break time wisely. If you are not able to keep track of your start/finish time, have someone be your timekeeper. When you complete the entire seven levels, with only 30-second breaks between levels, CONGRATS!

PHASE 2B:

Having completed Phase 2a, you now have the option of going on to Phase 2b, which means you'll do another round of Levels 1-7, increasing break times between levels from 30 to 45 seconds. I applaud you for accepting the challenge of taking on Phase 2b. This is difficult but you will have done it!

PHASE 3:

In Phase 3, Maintenance, I added a Bonus section inside the lower half of the chart for you, taking out the guesswork of trying to decide which levels to group together. I paired up two of the most effective levels that I believe will continually improve your body's ability to adapt. I have combined two of my levels to enhance your fitness routine, adding them three times a week for two weeks. You should aim to do this at the end of your workout. The reasons I would like you to select two exercises to incorporate at the end of each of your workouts are:

1. To help you complete each move with precision, even when fatigued. This will aid in building muscle memory and endurance.
2. If it's at the end of your workout, hopefully, you won't rush through the levels. As you focus on your chosen levels, I want you to feel the same body engagement and mindset you did when you were mastering each level.

After two weeks of those levels, pick two new ones and follow the same format. The Maintenance Phase will help you maintain a strong core in your game of play.

(Note: There will be a video available for purchase separately that demonstrates the setup of each level and total reps for the entire workout in one round!)

WHAT IF I THINK I CAN SKIP PHASE 1?

There are probably a few people out there who will be able to complete all seven levels the first time through. I would encourage another look at these levels, with special attention to body angle, control of movement, and timing of your breath. The end goal for each level is to make sure you always control the pace of your movement. If you're moving too fast through each level, you will not engage the correct muscle groups effectively and other muscle groups will try to compensate by taking over that movement. For each level, the aim is to focus on that specific muscle group to benefit your overall core strength.

Although the primary objective is to get through each level, even the path to mastery will yield benefits.

After you have mastered the seven levels and your sports season is approaching, I recommend you continue with Maintenance (two of my **METHOD** levels twice per week) even during your sports season. Keeping up with these specific exercises and unique movements will keep your abdominal muscles working in sync with each other. If you are in your prime sport season and unable to fit in Maintenance, begin at Level 1 and progress as directed until you can return to my **ENCORE METHOD**. During offseason training, I recommend reviewing all seven levels to refamiliarize your mind and body by doing all levels, paying close attention to body mechanics and form.

TIPS FOR THE HELPER/SPOTTER (especially for those who are new to core exercises):

1. Please remember that this may be difficult for some athletes, and they may be feeling a little frustrated during my core fitness program.

2. It will be imperative to always speak with a calm voice when cueing them.

3. At this level I would expect some athletes to feel unbalanced or stressed by the workout! Please remind them that if they lose their form or balance, they can take as long a break as needed to complete each side and the total amount of reps.

When struggling, remember these things:

- Have someone assist you in positioning (this may mean asking someone to place their hands on you for balance).
- Focus on your breath during the exercise. Take as many breaks as needed to get the prescribed number of repetitions.

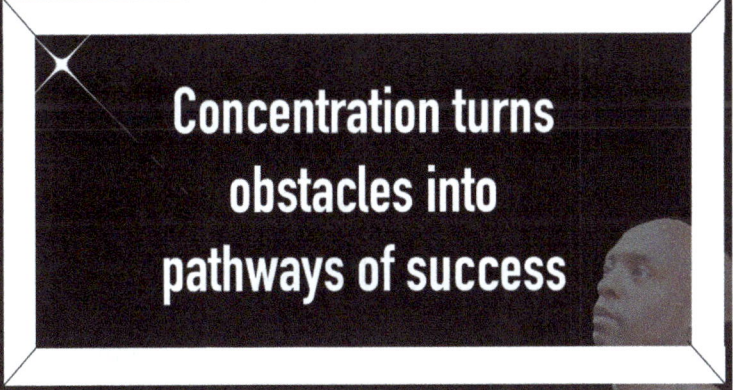

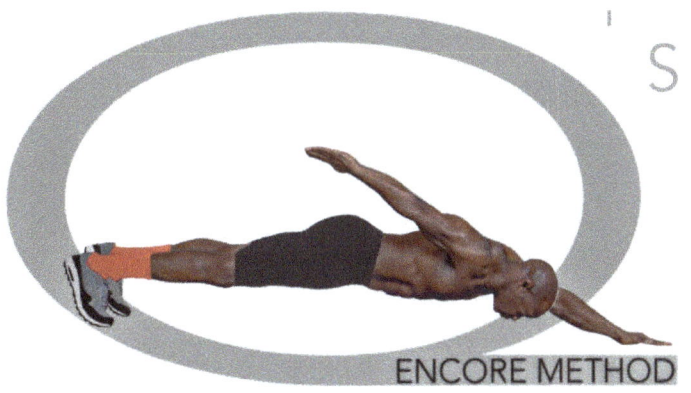

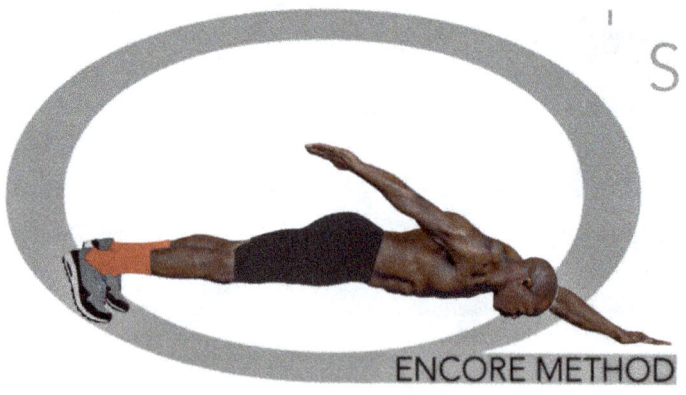

3.
Q'S ENCORE METHOD

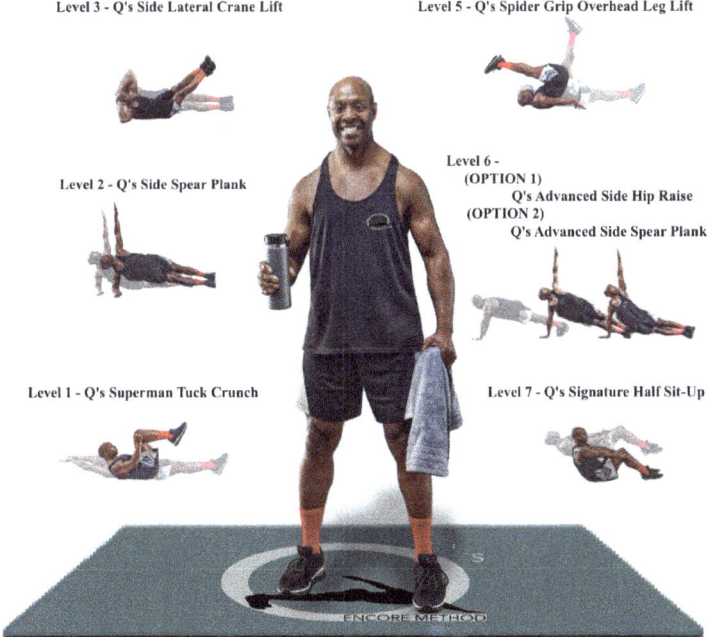

DISCOVER THE POWER of linking core muscles effectively with my 7 Levels program. Strengthen and engage your core like never before as you progress through each level. Achieve optimal results and unlock your body's true potential with this transformative approach.

Level 1 - Q's Superman Tuck Crunch

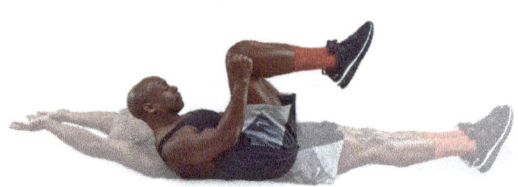

It's time to fire up the core! The starting position is on a mat with your arms extended overhead, palms up, legs extended, and feet pointed away from your body, as shown in Fig. 1.1, with heels resting on the ground. Feet should be slightly less than shoulder-width apart. Now, prepare your muscles for the movement to follow by elevating your head off the ground, taking a deep breath in, and bracing your abdominal muscles for the movement to follow.

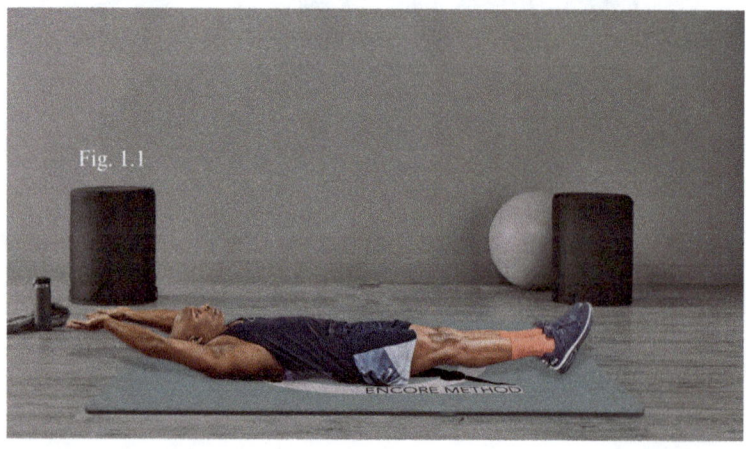

Fig. 1.1

In one slow, controlled movement, simultaneously contract your abdominals to raise your upper body. The goal is to contract your abdominal muscles enough so that you curl up into a tuck position. Your shoulder blades are slightly off the ground, making a space between your chin and chest (Fig. 1.2). Your arms should be about 90 degrees bent at the elbows and your hands in a light fist grip resting alongside your knees; the fists are a good cue for the stopping point of your knees. At this max contraction into the tuck position, pause briefly, then inhale and return to the starting position with arms and legs extended and head elevated as shown in Fig. 1.2. Tap (do not rest) your heels and begin your next repetition with an exhale. Repeat for 25 repetitions.

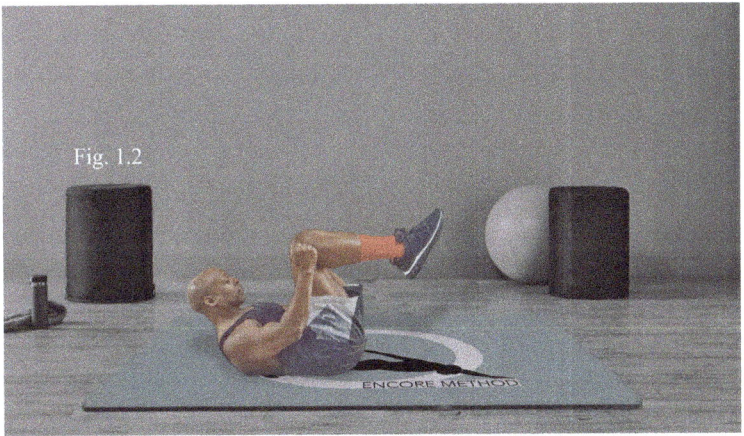

Fig. 1.2

TARGET MUSCLES: rectus abdominis, internal and external obliques

Level 2 - Q's Side Spear Plank

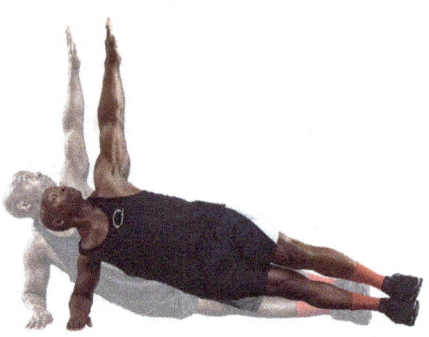

Mastering Q's Spear Side Plank will give you a competitive edge, allow you to take your workout or gameplay to a higher level, and help with foot agility and quickness.

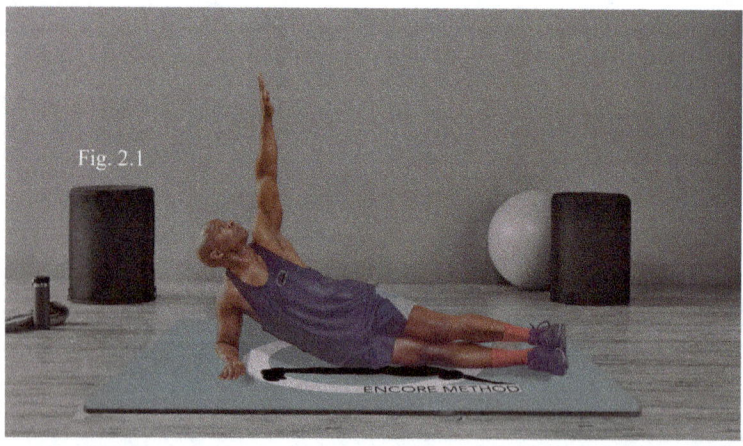

Fig. 2.1

Start on the mat in the position shown (Fig. 2.1), with weight bearing through your forearm, palm down, at a 90-degree angle, with feet stacked. Your body should be in a straight line from head to toe. During this exercise, maintain your raised arm in Q's Spear Formation. That means your hand is in a spear-like shape with fingers and thumb together. Rotate your head toward the raised hand, gazing past your fingertips. Maintain your head in this position throughout the exercise.

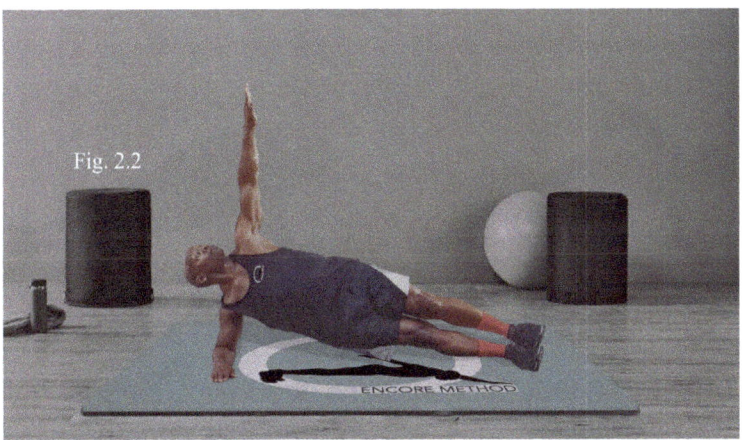

Fig. 2.2

Exhale as you raise your hip to the position shown in Fig. 2.2. It is important that your body is aligned with two straight lines: horizontal and vertical. The horizontal line goes through the shoulders, hips, and ankles (with feet stacked as shown). The vertical line goes through the supporting elbow and shoulders. Hold this position for 60 seconds, but don't hold your breath. Try to focus on normal breathing while maintaining this position. When the 60 seconds have been reached, slowly lower your hip to the floor. Quickly change to the opposite side and position yourself as shown in Fig 2.1 again, then move as instructed into the position shown in Fig. 2.2. Do not take a rest after the first side.

Supporting the body are deltoids (shoulder stabilizing muscles), gluteus medius, and gluteus minimus. Unlike in the traditional plank (Fig. 2.3), where either the hand is on the hip or alongside the body giving more support to stabilizing the position, in Q's Side Spear Plank the hand is extended upward and away from the body, forcing you to maintain your balance and focus.

Fig. 2.3

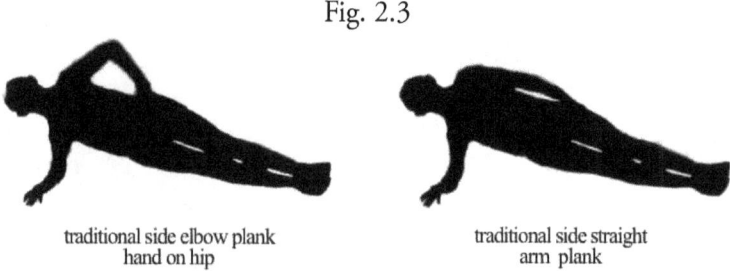

traditional side elbow plank hand on hip

traditional side straight arm plank

TARGET MUSCLES: transverse abdominis, internal and external obliques, latissimus dorsi, quadratus lumborum

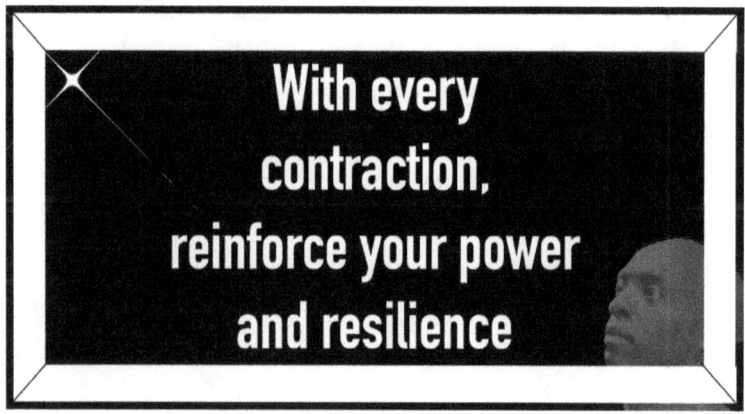

With every contraction, reinforce your power and resilience

Level 3 - Q's Side Lateral Crane Lift

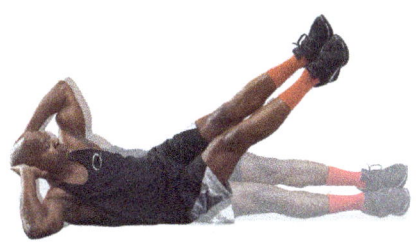

WOW, great that you have made it this far! Keep up the good work and stay focused. By utilizing slow and controlled movements, you are allowing your internal and external obliques to work in unison to raise and lower your legs together.

This next exercise will help with lateral control. It will improve your body's ability to make quick directional changes. Q's Side Lateral Crane Lifts prep the muscles to work together for these movements. This exercise also helps maintain your balance on uneven surfaces (e.g. incline, decline, or uneven slope of a hill) and helps you stay stable when standing, even when the surface is slippery.

Once again, positioning is key to progressing through this exercise. As you look closely at Fig. 3.1, pay attention to the position and angle. Your body should not be perpendicular to the floor but rolled back about 15 degrees. To obtain this angle, roll backward slightly off your hip bone and maintain this angle throughout the exercise (Fig. 3.2). Make sure your head is alongside the raised arm.

28 | Q's ENCORE METHOD

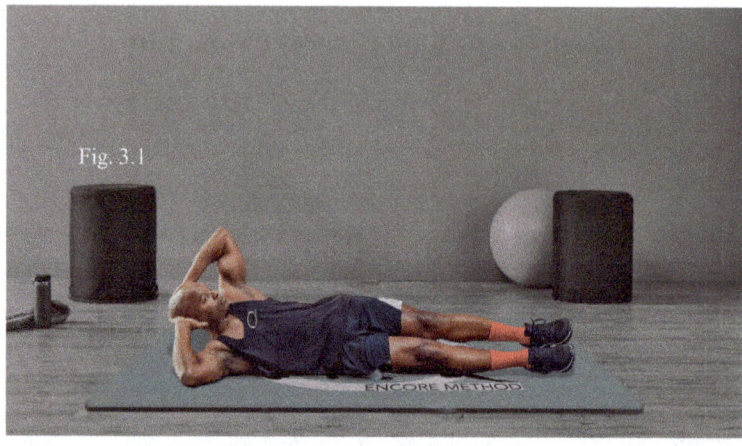

Fig. 3.1

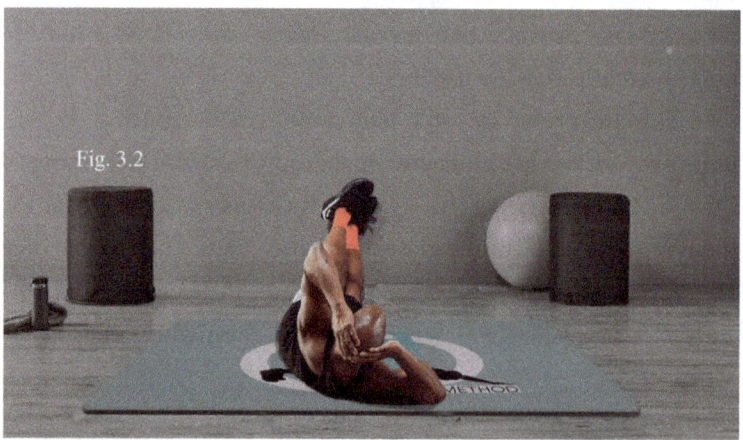

Fig. 3.2

    Keep legs pressed together at knees and ankles. Fig. 3.3 shows how both legs should be slightly bent, with feet stacked and pointed at an upright angle away from your body. Apply pressure through the supporting elbow and hip as you elevate your legs. Exhale as you lift, using your obliques, until your feet are about 2 feet off the floor, or stop when your heels reach your elevated elbow height. Inhale. Slowly lower back to the starting position with one side of the heel lightly tapping the ground. Repeat this cycle of lifting and lowering with a slow, controlled pace for 16 repetitions per side. This should be a constant cycle of lifting and lowering. Do not rest with the heel tap. The results of the movement will help stabilize the transverse abdominis and low back muscles.

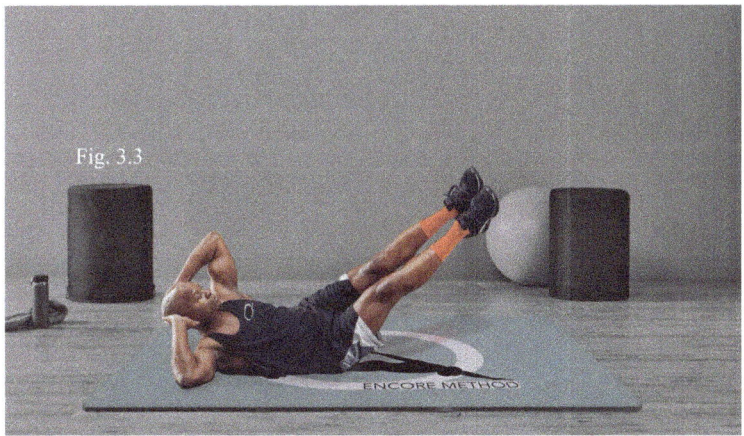

Fig. 3.3

TARGET MUSCLES: internal and external obliques, abductors and adductors

OKAY, FITNESS ENTHUSIASTS AND ATHLETES, HERE'S YOUR NEXT CORE CHALLENGE!

Level 4 - Q's Knee to Elbow Mountain Climber

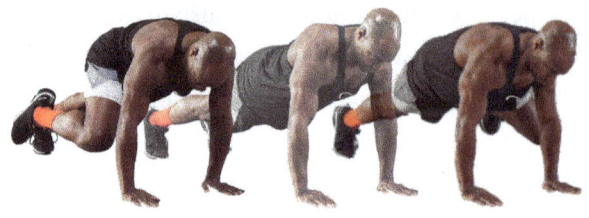

This exercise will help improve your balance and control and will aid in increasing your speed and endurance. When you are in the plank position, the traditional mountain climber exercise will drive your knees beneath your chest, mostly focusing on the rectus abdominis. Here, by driving your knees away from your body, towards your outer elbows, you will increase your endurance by engaging the quads, lower back, internal and external obliques, and hip flexors, employing more muscle groups. You will definitely feel it in your obliques! I believe Q's Knee to Elbow Mountain Climbers will improve your speed and acceleration.

Alternately driving each knee towards your elbow is considered one repetition. Thirty mountain climbers will surely increase your heart rate and your endurance. So what are you waiting for? Let's get after it!

Start in a push-up position with arms and legs straight, as pictured in Fig. 4.1. Make sure your hands and feet are shoulder-width apart and in line with your hands.

Take a look at Fig. 4.2 and note the position of the right knee. It is in line with the elbow and the toes are not in contact with the floor. Note that this is the fully flexed knee position in which you are driving each knee outside the body in the direction of the elbow on the same side. Keep your head in a neutral position and your gaze in front of your hands. When your right foot returns to the starting position, quickly transition as shown in Fig. 4.3 to the left side, driving the left knee in line with the left elbow and repeating for a total of 30 repetitions (combined right knee and left knee motion is one repetition).

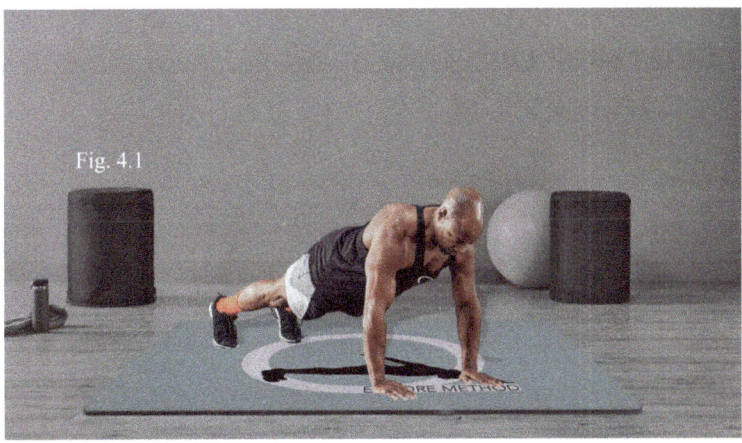

Fig. 4.1

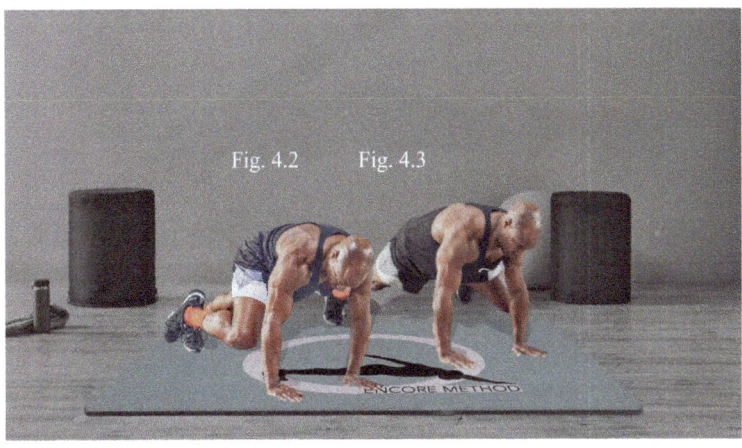

Fig. 4.2   Fig. 4.3

Meanwhile, make sure your hips are staying low; this will help avoid excessive weight shifting. Something to keep in mind is to try and establish your controlled pace by your sixth rep and try to maintain that pace for the remainder of the repetitions. Also, coordinate the exhale during the knee lift on each side. Quickly inhale as you transition to the other side. For this exercise, you will take smaller, quicker breaths.

TARGET MUSCLES: glutes, quads, abs, hamstrings, shoulders and triceps

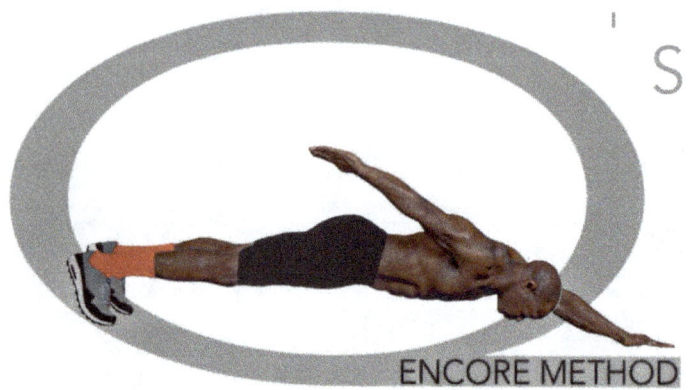

Level 5 - Q's Spider Grip Overhead Leg Lift

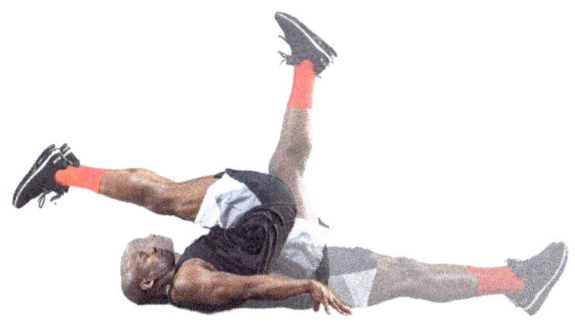

This exercise will vastly improve control between the quadriceps and your core and help initiate that quick burst of speed. When you begin that first quick step, your core should naturally engage, but it could be out of sync with that first step. This exercise helps connect the quads and core for acceleration. In everyday life, this helps with lifting and moving heavy objects, like furniture. This move will help mind and body naturally turn on core muscles to help you move something heavy, while also protecting your lower back.

While lying on your back, start with your head raised off the ground. Arms should be extended and elevated off the ground, alongside the body. Fingers should be in Spider Grip position as shown in Fig. 5.1. Fingertips are spread out and the furthest parts are in contact with the floor. Also, your legs should be completely straight, with your toes pointed away from your body. Pushing your fingertips into the floor and focusing on closing the gap between your lower back and the floor, will create the base of the body's crane (that is, the body from shoulder to hip). The crane provides the stability to control the movement needed next.

34 | Q's ENCORE METHOD

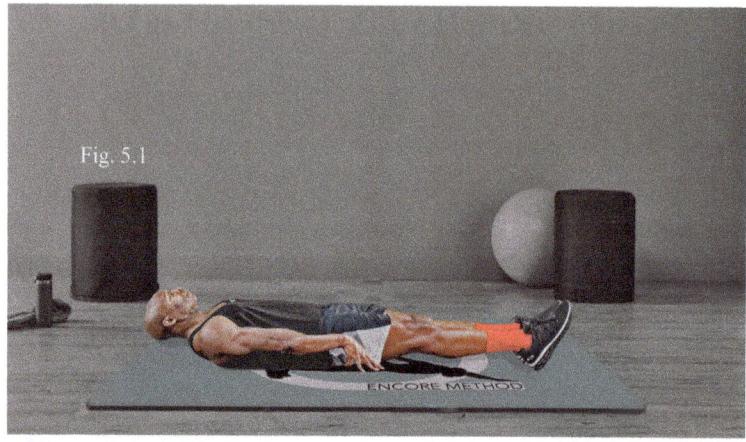

Fig. 5.1

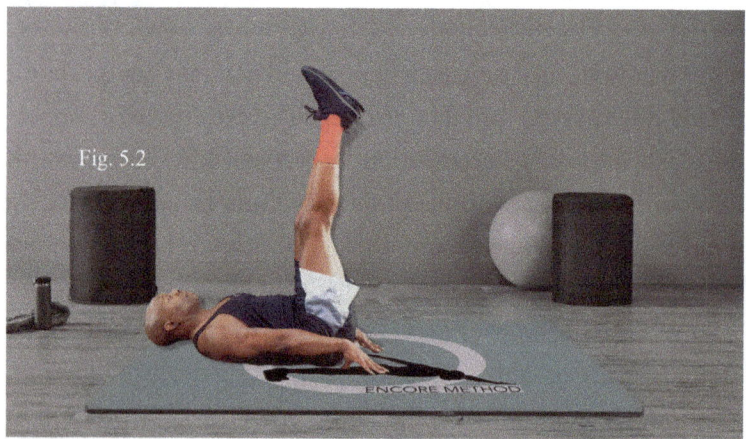

Fig. 5.2

As you initiate the leg lift to move to the position shown in Fig. 5.2, engage your abdominals by pressing your lower back into the ground, and then begin to exhale. Elevate your legs using your abdominals and hip flexors to bring them to a 90-degree angle as shown in Fig. 5.2. This is now our starting and ending position for Q's Spider Grip Overhead Leg Lift.

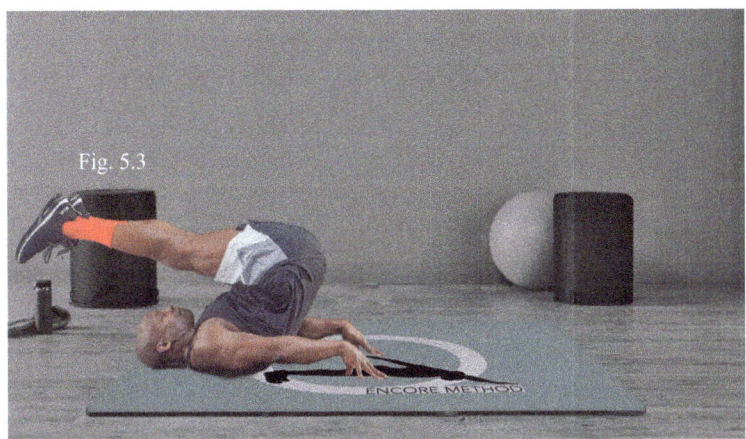

Fig. 5.3

Remember to keep your head elevated but relaxed, and your gaze straight up. Do a quick inhale and an exhale to reset, and then a full exhale as you move to Fig. 5.3. Your core is hoisting your feet up, beyond and over your head and as you move. Your head naturally lowers to the floor and despite its inclination to lift up, it should remain on the floor for the repetitions. This should be a controlled lowering of the feet over the head to no less than one foot off the ground. Pause for a moment to maintain control. Then, as you undo this position, *inhale,* as you lower your back down to the floor. Once your back is completely flat against the floor, make sure your legs stay at 90 degrees and your toes are pointed upward. This is the end of one rep, but don't rest here. Begin your *exhale* as you hoist your legs again. Push into those fingertips to begin the lift. Complete these movements for 12 repetitions.

TARGET MUSCLES: Arm and finger extensors, erector spinae, quadratus lumborum, rectus abdominis, internal and external obliques and transverse abdominis

Level 6 - (OPTION 1) Q's Advanced Side Hip Raise
(OPTION 2) Q's Advanced Side Spear Plank

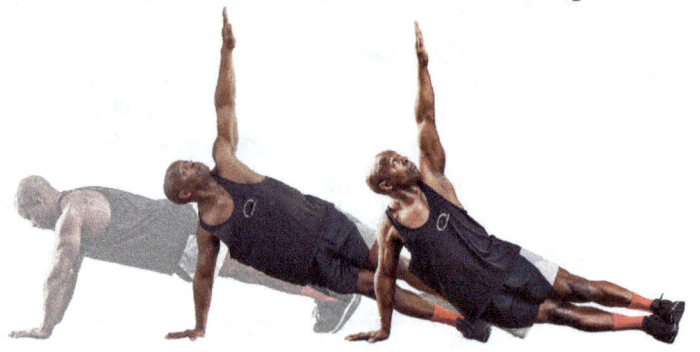

OPTION 1

With Level 6, you will be given two Options. Option 1, Q's Advanced Side Hip Raise, will be more difficult because it involves lowering and raising your hip while maintaining your balance. When starting off with this exercise, make sure to focus on the description of the setup to master it. Start out in a push-up position with your hands shoulder-width apart, the palms of your hands right in front of the base of the shoulders, fingers spread apart, and feet together (Fig. 6.1).

Moving into the next position (Fig. 6.2), fingers should be spread apart on the support hand on the mat and pointing away from your body. This exercise will be done first on one side and then on the other. For foot placement, keep feet close together during this setup position. While maintaining hand position, move into Q's Spear Formation by turning your body sideways, extending your non-support arm into an upright position, and keeping your fingers together. Your head should be turned to gaze up at your fingertips, remaining that way throughout the movement.

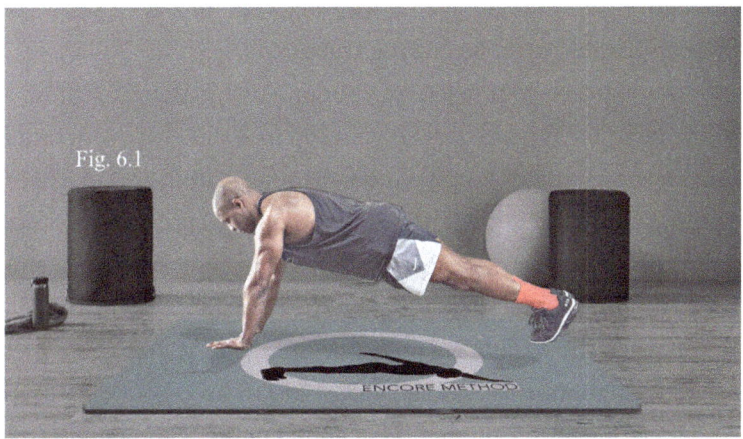

Fig. 6.1

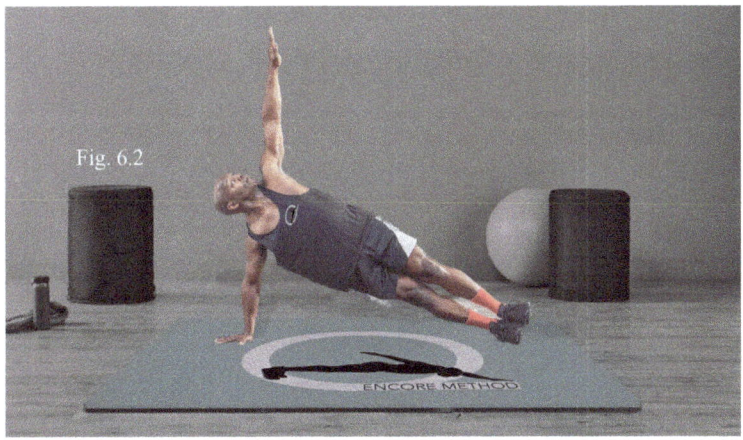

Fig. 6.2

Now relax your shoulder, hip, and knee while lowering your hip as close as possible to the floor. Engaging your abdominals will help you control your balance when raising and lowering your body. Inhale as you lower your hip and exhale as you raise your hip. The ultimate goal is to lower your hip as close to the floor as possible without making contact.

To increase your range of motion in this exercise, allow a gentle bend in your legs and let your top foot slide over your other foot, as shown in Fig. 6.3. Keep the spear formation arm in a fixed position throughout the downward and upward movement. Since your knees were bent during the downward movement, remember to re-engage your quadriceps on the rising phase to assist with returning to the straight leg position. Complete 12 repetitions per side. Throughout this exercise, remember to keep your eyes fixed on a spot on the ceiling that is beyond your spear formation.

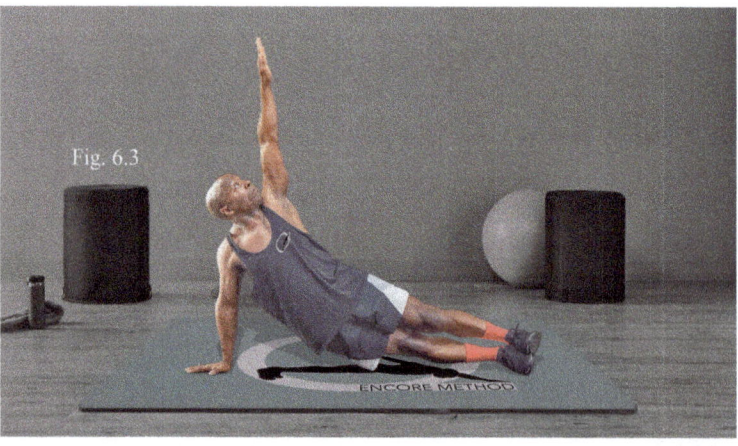

Fig. 6.3

Q'S ENCORE METHOD | 39

OPTION 2

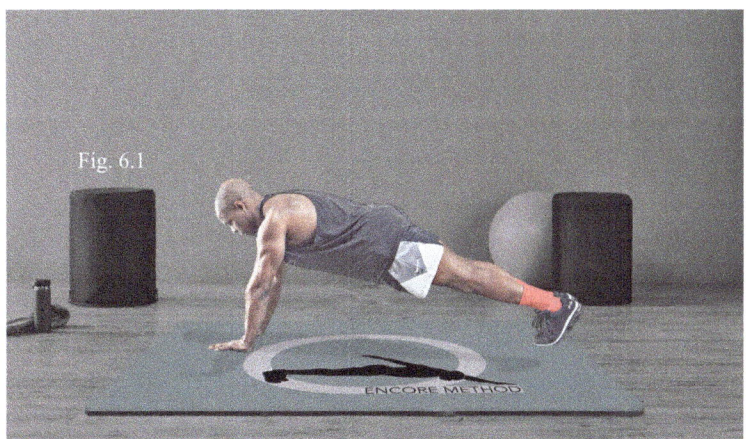

Fig. 6.1

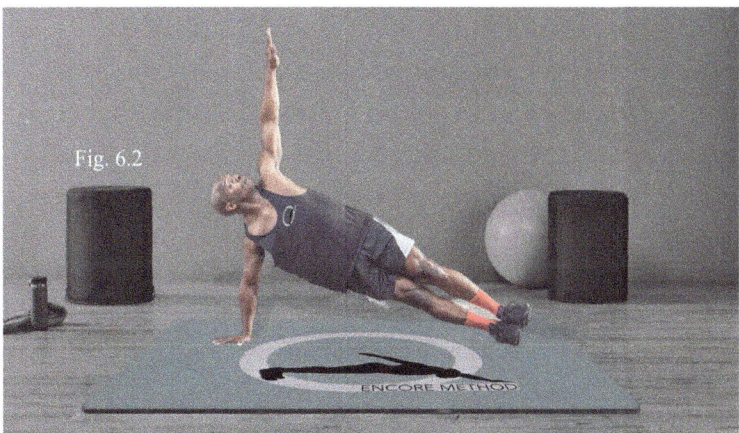

Fig. 6.2

Fig. 6.2, Option 2 is an alternative for those who struggle with the more difficult movement in Option 1, or who may have a prior lower back stress injury. Option 2 will help protect and stabilize your core muscles. In this alternative option, you will need to hold Q's Side Spear Plank (Level 2) for 60 seconds without loss of balance. For both options, it is important to keep your feet together even when rotating to the other side of the body. Duplicate the same position on the opposite side of the body without stopping, holding for 60 seconds.

I created this exercise to help with balance, stability, and side-to-side movements. When playing a contact sport such as football, hockey, lacrosse, etc., this exercise will help you withstand the impact of a collision that targets your obliques and lower back. Additionally, it can help you maintain whole-body awareness while responding to contact from an opponent, and also enhance speed and agility. Although Q's Advanced Side Hip Raises are similar to exercise Option 2, this version involves a static hold, while Option 1 requires repeated contractions.

TARGET MUSCLES: deltoid, transverse abdominis, internal and external obliques, latissimus dorsi, quadratus lumborum, tensor fasciae latae, gluteus medius and minimis, adductor longus

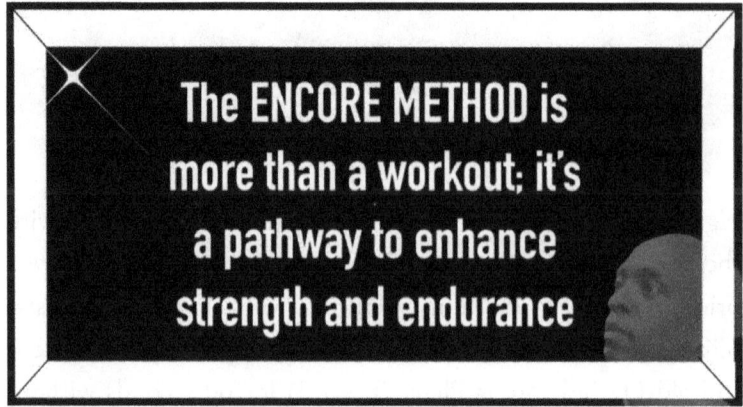

Level 7 - Q's Signature Half Sit-Up

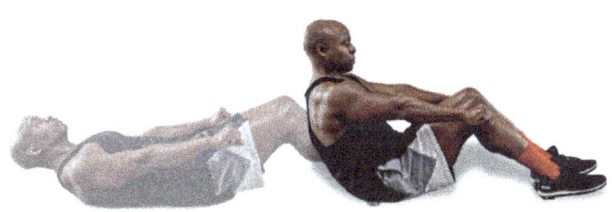

A full sit-up can put extra pressure on your lower back and tailbone. Limiting the range of motion from the full sit-up targets the rectus abdominis more effectively throughout the movement. As I tell my clients, this exercise may look easy, but don't be fooled! Q's Signature Half Sit-Ups will create endless muscle contractions in your rectus abdominis. Believe me, you will feel the burn! This unique exercise will help contract your abdomen more effectively. Often the abs relax at the beginning and end of a traditional sit-up. A strong rectus abdominis can aid with speed, quickness, and agility.

Begin by lying down on the floor on your back, with your knees angled slightly wider than 90 degrees. Your feet should be about 1.5 to 2 feet away from your glutes. Make sure your head is elevated off the floor and in a neutral position. Hold your arms up outside your knees as shown in Fig. 7.1, keeping your hands in a light fist grip, palms facing downward. Your back should be raised enough that your shoulder blades are also elevated slightly off the floor.

42 | Q's ENCORE METHOD

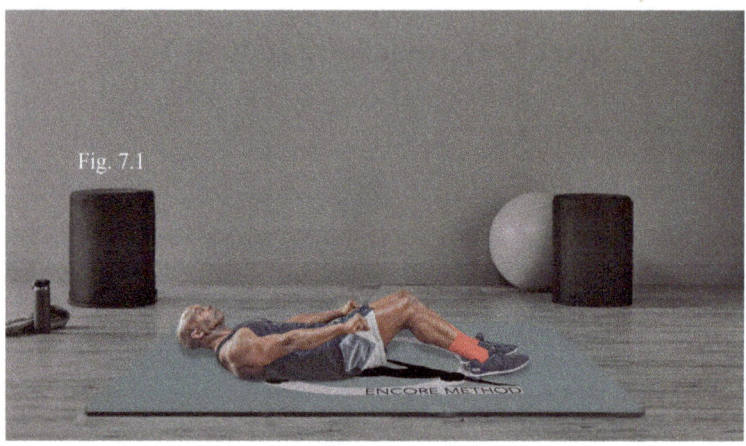

Fig. 7.1

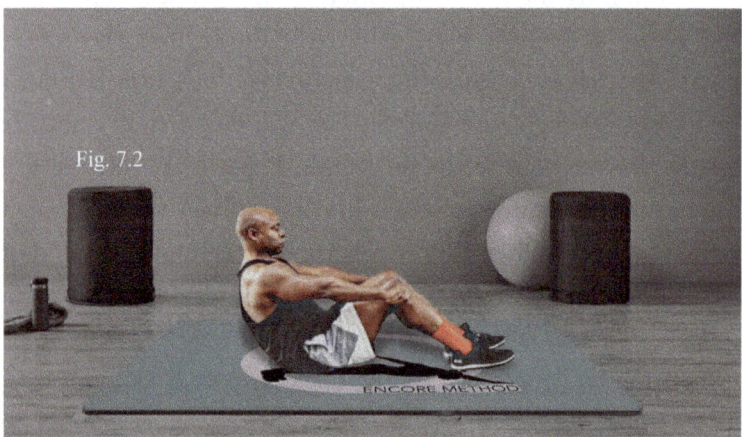

Fig. 7.2

There are two separate movements that initiate the transition from Fig. 7.1 to Fig. 7.2: (1) keep your arms extended, and (2) create the lift with your mid and lower rectus abdominis. To initiate this upright movement, first make sure your arms are straight and elevated on either side of your body, hands in a light fist grip in the direction of the knees, palms facing downward. Then exhale and begin to lift with the abdominals (Fig. 7.1). Continue to lift and reach until your fists align with the knees. Keep your chin away from your chest throughout the movement. Remember, the motion is controlled: do not swing your arms for momentum.

Also, make sure heels remain in contact with the floor and keep your knees at greater than 90 degrees of flexion. Keep this movement short and precise (this is not a full sit-up), exhaling on the upright movement, inhaling on the downward movement. Lift up slowly, then lower slowly until your shoulder blades come in contact with the floor. Keep your head and neck elevated throughout this exercise. Pay special attention to the fists, making sure they don't extend past the knee joints. Complete 20 repetitions.

TARGET MUSCLES: rectus abdominis, transverse abdominis, internal and external obliques

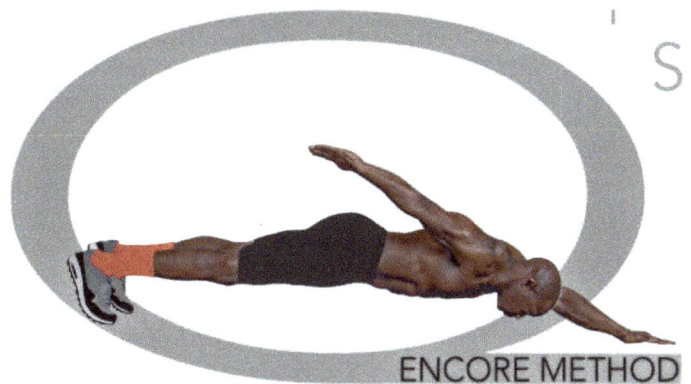

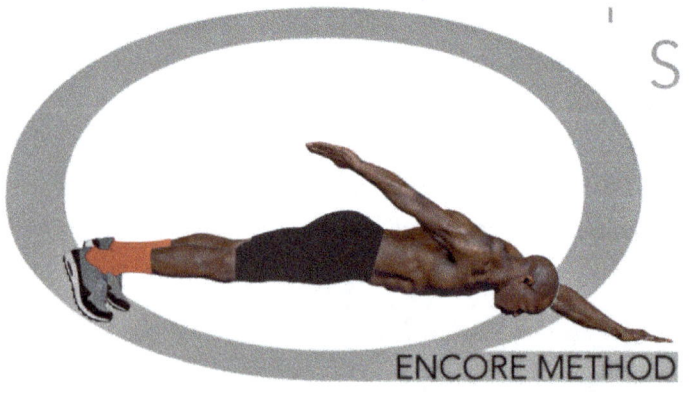

4.
Q'S ENCORE METHOD INTO ACTION

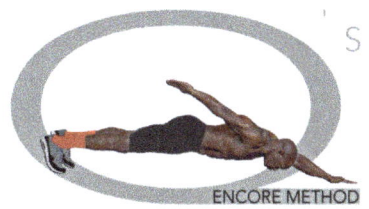

NOW YOU'RE READY to embark' on an exhilarating fitness journey with **Q's ENCORE METHOD**—a program designed to challenge your limits, unlock your hidden strength, and elevate your fitness game to new heights. The Progress Chart in Chapter 2 serves as a roadmap to your transformation, signaling the next phase of your evolution after conquering the initial seven exercises. As you delve deeper into the world of **Q's ENCORE METHOD**, each exercise becomes a steppingstone toward a stronger, fitter, and more resilient version of yourself.

Embrace the thrill of the challenge as you push past boundaries and discover the untapped potential within you. With each movement, you will feel the surge of accomplishment and empowerment, knowing that every step brings you closer to your fitness goals. Fuel your determination with the knowledge that every sweat session is a step forward on the path to greatness.

Prepare for an adventure that is both rewarding and fun, where the joy of progress intertwines with the satisfaction of overcoming obstacles. Stay engaged and motivated as you navigate through the phases of the program, feeling the exhilaration of growth and transformation with each successful workout. Embrace the journey with an open heart and a fearless spirit, knowing that the challenges ahead will only make the victories sweeter. Get ready to push yourself, have fun, and experience the thrill of unlocking your full potential with **Q's ENCORE METHOD**.

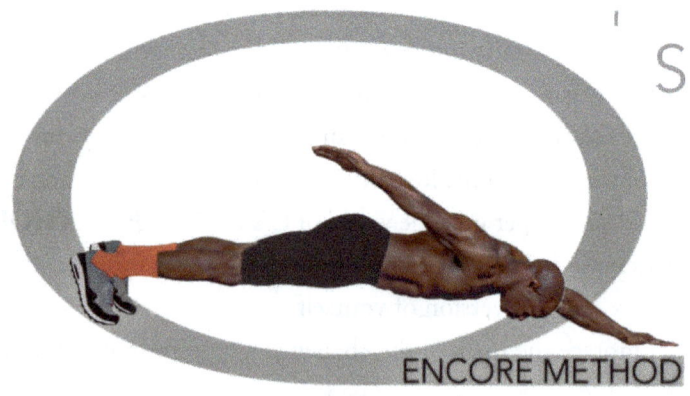

BONUS SECTION:
Q RECOMMENDS THREE ESSENTIAL CORE STRETCHES

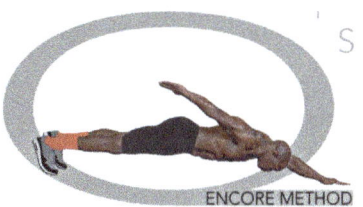

After each workout, I recommend the following three stretches:

1. YOGA COBRA STRETCH

The primary focus of this stretch is to release tension in the rectus abdominis and hip flexors, shoulders, and low back. This is one of my favorite stretches.

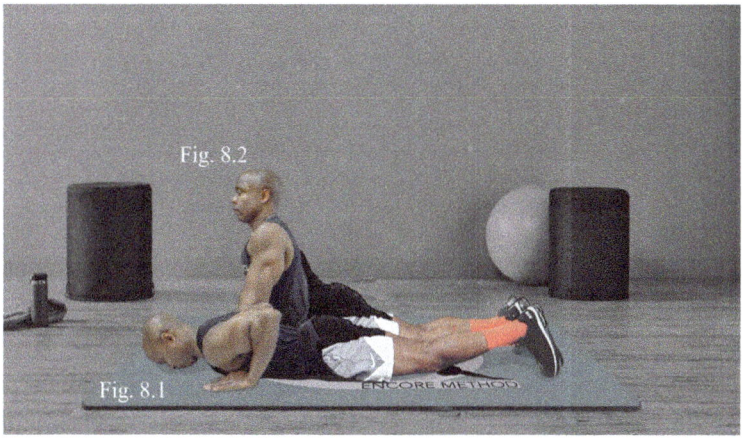

Begin lying on the floor face-down, but with your head elevated off the floor, and elbows and hands close to the body. Knees and feet should be no greater than shoulder-width apart (Fig. 8.1). Maintain lower body (knees and feet) in this position for this stretch. Be sure to inhale and exhale normally while in this position. Start off with an exhale while you push into the floor to extend your arms. Maintain your head in neutral alignment as you move from the position in Fig. 8.1 to Cobra position as shown in Fig. 8.2. Try to fully extend your arms as this will increase the stretch in your abdominals and hip flexors, listening to your body and stopping when you feel a stretch, but not to the point of discomfort. Hold for 10 seconds while breathing at a normal rate.

2. YOGA CHILD'S POSE AND LATERAL STRETCH

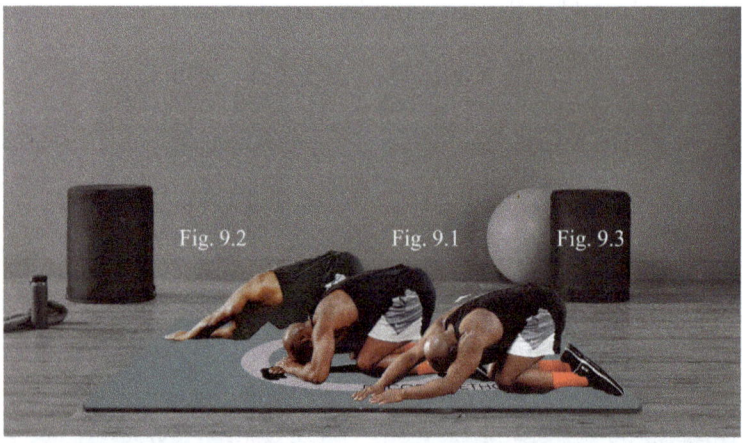

Now, you will flow into the next position, Child's Pose. As you move out of the Cobra Pose, try to sit back on your heels while inhaling. Be sure to space your knees and feet hip-width apart (Fig. 9.1). The goal is to sit back between your heels as close to the floor as possible. This will depend on the level of flexibility in your lower back and quadriceps. Also, move your hands back towards your body to about a foot from your knees and place the palm of one hand on top of the other, resting your forehead on the back of your hands. Exhale when you have reached your limit of flexibility. Inhale and exhale with slow, controlled breathing in this resting position. During the inhale, you should feel your rib cage and lower back expand. Make sure your body is relaxed with each exhale. Hold this stretch for 20 seconds. Overall, this is a holistic, relaxing body movement, but the depth of the stretch will be unique to each person based on their lower back range of motion.

To begin the next part of this stretch, start by inhaling while elevating your head, then exhaling as you slide your hands to the right (Fig. 9.2). Hold this position, relax your head on the floor while slowly inhaling and exhaling for 10-15 seconds. Repeat the movement on your other side (Fig. 9.3). Complete two sets making sure to stretch both sides evenly.

3. Q'S KNEELING OBLIQUES STRETCH

From a standing position, lower your left knee to the ground, left foot and right knee less that hip-width apart. Raise your right arm into Q's Spear Formation with your palm facing away from your body (Fig. 10.1) and your left arm resting alongside your thigh. Be sure to stabilize your hips directly over your knees at the beginning and when moving with the stretch. You will do three things at once as you start the movement: (1) (Fig. 10.1) reach overhead, (2) begin to exhale, and (3) slide your hand down the side of your leg. This exhale should last the duration of the downward movement. Go as far as possible while maintaining a comfortable side stretch and still keeping the alignment of the hips, knees, and feet. Inhale as you return to the starting position. Keep your arm bent overhead during the six controlled repetitions. Then duplicate these steps on the other side.

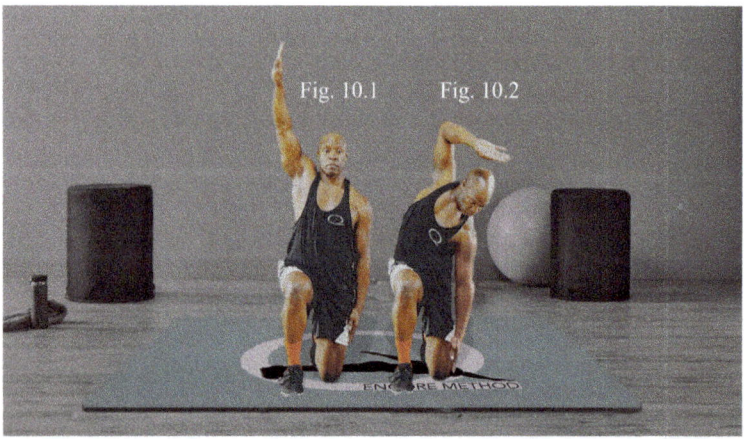

If you want a deeper stretch of your obliques, try touching your fingertips to the floor (see Fig. 10.2). The goal is six repetitions. Stay on one side before stretches and all reps are completed. Remember to inhale each time as you lift back up to the starting position. Also, this is a "dynamic" stretch so do not rest in any one position - try to keep moving at a controlled pace.

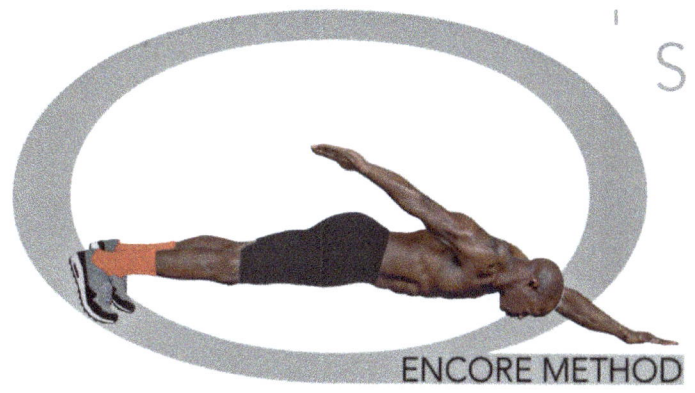

THE STEALTH PLANK™ is Quincy Kidd's signature pose—a visual representation of control, alignment, and mastery within **Q's ENCORE METHOD**. It symbolizes the full-body tension, focus, and strength that athletes and everyday individuals strive for.

This position is not meant to be trained or replicated by everyone—it stands as a personal mastery marker, a reminder that elite form begins with disciplined core control.

THE STEALTH PLANK™ is part of Q's branding and philosophy, not a required movement in his training system.

It's a symbol—not a standard. A reminder of where strength begins, and how stillness can speak louder than motion.

CONCLUSION

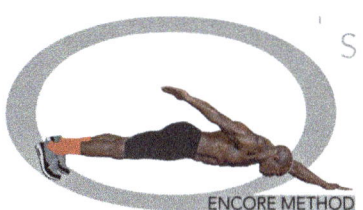

I HOPE YOU HAVE FOUND Q's ENCORE METHOD very useful, entertaining, engaging, and fun.

I appreciate your effort and time commitment to mastering my creative core strength exercises. If you have completed all seven exercises without losing your balance or form, I congratulate you! You are AWESOME and I believe in you. Your teammates and coaches will notice the difference in your level of play! Also, you will achieve an increase in overall body control. With the completion of my **METHOD**, your endurance will increase. Additionally, you will have the mindset and body awareness to adapt to quick, unexpected movements with stability and balance.

I'd also like to say "thank you so much" for the purchasing of my book. I hope it has been a great experience learning how important range of motion, body positioning, and alignment are to achieving that connection within your body. I hope you felt that some of these exercises were challenging to you. This experience might be different from anything you have done before, and I appreciate that you dove in and believed in the result. I have seen this commitment pay off in a higher level of play in many of my clients. With continued practice of the routine, you will see improvement in speed, power, foot agility, finesse, and confidence.

CONNECT WITH ODIS "QUINCY" KIDD III
For personalized training, speaking engagements, or any inquiries, feel free to get in touch:

Email: q@quincykiddcpt.com
Website: www.quincykiddcpt.com
Instagram: @quincykiddcpt
Facebook: @quincykiddcpt
Linkedin: @quincykiddcpt

ACKNOWLEDGMENTS

The iconic logo image—my signature pose known as *The Stealth Plank*™—was captured by **Lorn Spolter**, whose lens brought stillness and strength to life.

The front cover photo and one additional interior image were photographed and expertly retouched by **Jessica Simpson**, whose creative vision elevated the visual impact of this project.

All warm-up and movement images throughout the 7 Levels of training were photographed by **Jeff and Sandra Burt** of **Eclipse Creative**—thank you for your precision and professionalism.

Most importantly, I extend heartfelt thanks to **Joyce Simmons** for her strong editing support, and to the incredible team at **Columbus Publishing Lab**, whose skillful layout, design, and tone editing helped elevate this book to a polished, professional standard.

PERSONAL NOTE

To everyone who stood behind me during this journey, your encouragement, support, and belief helped shape this book from an idea into reality. I have friends, family, and clients who have been waiting patiently for this book to surface—and it's because of your consistent belief in my vision that I never stopped pushing forward.

I'm especially grateful to the fellow personal trainers who supported me early on—those who recognized the uniqueness of my method and reminded me that it truly delivers results. Your encouragement confirmed that this system needed to be shared with the world.

Through every challenge, I've leaned on my faith and the purpose God placed in my heart. This project represents more than movement—it's a statement of purpose, growth, and resilience. Thank you for helping me bring it to life.

"Commit to the Lord whatever you do, and He will establish your plans."
—Proverbs 16:3

BEST REGARDS,
ODIS QUINCY KIDD III

www.ingramcontent.com/pod-product-compliance
Lightning Source LLC
Chambersburg PA
CBHW060033040426
42333CB00042B/2416